MW01413418

Crohn's Disease and Colitis: Hidden Triggers and Symptoms

Artour Rakhimov

Disclaimer

The content provided herein is for information purposes only and not intended to diagnose, treat, cure or prevent cystic fibrosis or any other chronic disease. Always consult your doctor or health care provider before making any medical decisions). The information herein is the sole opinion of Dr. Artour Rakhimov and does not constitute medical advice. These statements have not been evaluated by Ontario Ministry of Health. Although every effort has been made to ensure the accuracy of the information herein, Dr. Artour Rakhimov accepts no responsibility or liability and makes no claims, promises, or guarantees about the accuracy, completeness, or adequacy of the information provided herein and expressly disclaims any liability for errors and omissions herein.

TABLE OF CONTENTS

Introduction

Contemporary books, internet sources and articles on IBD (inflammatory bowel disease), including books written by doctors and nutritionists, are full of myths and fantasies about causes and solutions to this health problem. IBD includes Crohn's disease and ulcerative colitis.

These are the most stubborn and difficult-to-treat digestive problems. At the present moment, most people with Crohn's disease require surgical intervention during their lifetime. There is no known cure for ulcerative colitis, and popular therapies may only reduce some symptoms of ulcerative colitis. This book focuses on these, most difficult conditions.

As a result of popular treatment methods, people are mainly busy with endless changes in their diet and the daily use of probiotics and other supplements. These treatment programs are sometimes sprinkled with ideas of better chewing, more exercise and other lifestyle changes. Typical success rates for most methods are virtually never reported since they are usually much less than 50% in the short run. In the long run, since there are no criteria for normal or good digestion, many of the recovered people will get the same and sometimes other symptoms some weeks or months later.

There are simply no books and internet resources that provide even a list of specific signs of normal digestive health. These signs do exist, and they include such factors that are virtually never mentioned in the medical literature or sources related to alternative medicine. For example, a person with normal digestive health does not require any toilet paper due to the absence of soiling (i.e., no residue is left on the anus after a bowel movement). Also, bowel movements are regular, and the feces do not produce any odor and do not leave marks on the toilet bowl.

If someone has a GI problem (such as inflammatory bowel disease), they always require use of toilet paper and the degree of soiling generally correlates with the severity of their digestive problem. Most ordinary people require toilet paper as well. This is an indicator of their poor GI health.

A person with normal digestion is able to hold up to 1 liter (4.2 cups) of urine in the urinary bladder, while modern sources do not even mention frequent urination with reduced urinary volume as one of the key symptoms of active digestive problems, such as Crohn's disease or ulcerative colitis.

Normal digestive health is also manifested in the absence of a tongue coating: scraping the tongue does not yield any white or yellow thick coating. Normal digestion means that there is no need to regularly or perpetually consume pounds of yogurt, probiotics, and/or any other fermented foods due to the continuous presence of good bacteria in the gut since the healthy immune system does not allow pathogens to reside on the surface of the gut and form biofilms.

All mentioned and other signs of good digestion relate to normalization of gut flora and the absence of pathological microbial films on the surface of the small intestine. This is another key topic that is rarely discussed. Formation of biofilms by pathogens is the norm in cases of inflammatory bowel disease. These biofilms prevent absorption of nutrients and pollute the body with toxins.

Soiling has a very simple cause directly related to biofilms. In fact, soiling indicates a dominance of common pathogens in the gut, such as Candida Albicans and H. Pylori. In conditions of low body O2, pathogens are able to survive and even thrive on the mucosal lining of the GI system. Biofilms are created by "sticky" pathogens, while good bacteria, which favor the absence of soiling, are unable to adhere to the surface of the gut. (The same sticky pathogens make one's stool greasy and leave marks on the walls of the toilet bowl.)

When people improve their body-O2 content up to the medical norm (40 seconds for the body-oxygen test), regardless of their initial health states and existing digestive problems, they naturally acquire these and other signs of good digestive health. However, people with IBD are not able to increase their body-O2 content (it remains at about 20-25 seconds) due to digestive flare-ups or acute exacerbations. This happens due to hidden triggers that chronically keep the gut inflamed.

Therefore, it is crucial to find out and address all those triggers and lifestyle factors that make their health worse.

You can consume tons of super foods and supplements, observe the most stringent diets for years, practice yoga and many other techniques for many hours every day, but if your body-O2 content remains unchanged, then the state of your immune system, blood flow and oxygenation of the GI organs, and overall health will also remain unchanged. If you increase your body O2 up to 40 or more seconds, then you will naturally acquire the main signs of good (or normal) digestive health.

1. Good and poor digestive health

In this chapter, we are going to focus on general topics related to good digestive health. We will consider common symptoms and signs of poor digestive health, causes of digestive problems and falre-ups in modern people, and expected effects of increased body oxygenation on digestive problems and restoration of normal digestive health even if you have Crohn's disease or colitis.

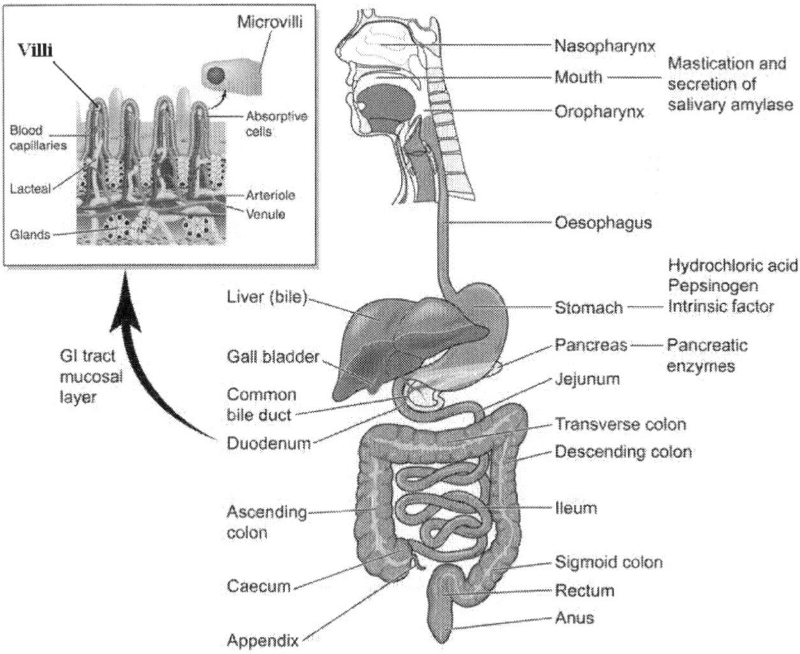

1.1 Common symptoms of digestive problems

Common symptoms of GI problems are known and described in many books and other information sources. These symptoms can appear within hours after meals, or can even be triggered by other factors (that are discussed later). These GI symptoms include:

- *bloating*

- *belching*

- *flatulence*

- *diarrhea*

- *constipation*

- *fullness*

- *nausea*

- *rectal itching.*

There are many additional symptoms that are usually ignored by most doctors. However, these symptoms are important due to their intimate relationship with digestive health. This relates to such symptoms as tongue coating, frequent urination, constantly moist nose, ear buzzing, cold feet, unquenchable thirst, degree of soiling (how much toilet paper is required), changes in water color in the toilet bowl, shape and consistency of stool, and others.

Digestive symptoms that require medical attention

- *rectal bleeding*

- *anemia*

- *lack of appetite*

- *significant weight loss*

- *vomiting*

- *middle of the night abdominal pain and cramping.*

1.2 Signs of good digestive health (absence of digestive problems)

Normal digestive health can be described as the ability of the GI tract to produce digestive enzymes, efficiently absorb nutrients, prevent growth of pathogens, recycle useful nutrients and chemicals, and eliminate toxins and unwanted substances.

Good digestive health also can be identified by the presence of good GI flora in the gut with a prevalence of friendly bacteria and absence of biofilms. People with less than 30 seconds for the morning body-oxygen test (or more than 90% of modern people) usually naturally harbor pathogens in the gut. Abnormal GI flora is manifested in numerous signs, some of which are summarized in the Table below.

Parameter	Ideal GI health	Diarrhea	Constipation
Tongue coating	None	Thick, yellow or white	Thick, yellow or white
Transition time	24-48 hours	Less than 24 hours	More than 48 hours
Regularity of bowel movements	Yes	No	No
Shape of feces	Well-formed regular sausages	Flaky, greasy, and irregular	Hardened and dried in the front part and soft and greasy at the end
Water in the sink	Remains clean	Does not remain clean	May remain clean
Marks on the sink wall	None	Very likely	Possible
Residue on the anus ("soiling effect")	None	Yes	Yes
Toilet paper	Unnecessary	Required	Required
Gas	Little or odorless	Likely; offensive	Likely; offensive
Additional signs	None	Possible flatulence, belching, burping, GERD	Possible flatulence, belching, burping, GERD

Body-oxygen content is the key factor that defines the strength of the immune system and predetermines one's digestive health. When the body oxygenation in the morning is about 30-35 seconds or more, the immune system starts to successfully reject pathogens from the mucosal surfaces of the large and small intestines and other GI organs. This leads to rapid disappearance of digestive problems. Numerous positive changes indicate changes towards the ideal digestive health.

On the other hand, poor digestive health is manifested in various unpleasant symptoms and effects described in the Table above.

Due to the presence of inflamed villi and GI biofilms, many breathing students get stuck at about 20-25 s for the morning body-oxygen test even if they try to do more physical and breathing exercises. The key reason of their lowered CPs is biochemical stress due to inflammation and pathogens in the GI system. This abnormal state of the GI system can exist due to low body O2 (less than 20 s) and/or due to harmful stimuli or triggers that leads to digestive flare-ups (or exacerbations). These triggers include hidden factors such as gluten or dairy products in diet, wrong types of physical exercise, wrong breathing exercises, and many others. There are in total several dozen adverse factors that are important to know and address in order to ensure GI recovery.

Without getting over 30 s for body oxygenation, it is very difficult or sometimes impossible to permanently solve many GI problems. However, chronic GI flare-ups drive the CP down to about 20-25 s or even smaller numbers. This leads to the formation of the vicious circle that is impossible to break unless a person identifies all these factors and makes and carries out a comprehensive plan to address them.

Increased urination and reduced volumes of urine per toilet trip are additional signs of poor GI health. A healthy bladder can hold up to about 1 liter of urine. When there are large structural abnormalities in the large or small intestines (such as inflammation, tumors, diverticula, and so on), the person cannot hold more than 500 ml of urine and has more frequent trips to the washroom/toilet. During flare-ups or when digestive problems are more severe, this amount can drop down to as low as 200-300 ml or even less.

Increased frequency of urination and small urinary volumes can be signs of prostatitis, UTI (urinary tract infections) and some other health problems. However, for most people with digestive problems, which are originated in bowels, frequent urination is a symptom that indicates the presence and degree of abnormalities (e.g., inflammation).

When the small intestine is involved, apart from increased urination and soiling, it is common to experience additional symptoms such as:

- *ear buzzing*

- *cold feet*

- *unquenchable thirst after meals or due to other triggers*

- *constantly moist nose.*

Furthermore, these symptoms are also sensitive to and reflect one's current GI health. These symptoms will be discussed in more detail later.

Since most people have less than 25 seconds for the body-oxygen test, intestinal dysbiosis and the soiling effect (a need to use toilet paper) are very common, indicating poor digestive health. Virtually all people who get over 50 seconds for the body-oxygen test testify that they do not need toilet paper anymore (or some of them may say that they have very little soiling, but this can happen only due to insufficient chewing). As a result, the no-soiling effect appears naturally due to retraining of the automatic breathing pattern for people with high body-O2 content.

1.3 Causes of digestive problems and poor GI health

Causes of poor digestive health are numerous. They are discussed throughout this book. We need to understand that there are differences between fundamental causes (such as low body-O2 content) and triggers (or technical mistakes, such as eating foods that irritate the gut, insufficient chewing, and so forth).

By fundamental causes I mean those primary physiological factors that make one's digestive recovery impossible. These factors include reduced blood flow (or perfusion) and oxygen supply to GI organs, and a suppressed state of the immune system. When the immune system functions normally and the GI organs have normal oxygenation and blood circulation, there are conditions for digestive recovery since the immune system will not allow the pathogens to form biofilms, which prevent absorption of nutrients and generate toxins that suppress the immune system and reduce body oxygenation. Normal immunity also includes the ability of the body to eliminate abnormalities such as inflammation, tumors, diverticula, strictures and so forth.

Virtually each and every person with digestive problems has reduced body-O2 content. The cause of reduced body-O2 content and, therefore, the main cause of digestive problems is abnormal or ineffective automatic breathing. There are 3 fundamental causes of low body O2: mouth breathing, chest breathing and chronic hyperventilation (the main cause that triggers 2 previous causes).

When blood flow to vital organs is below the norm and the body-O2 content is reduced (below 20 seconds for the body-O2 test described below), the immune system gets suppressed due to free radicals caused by cell hypoxia. This is the case, at least for early morning hours, for more than 90% of people. However, this was not the case with ordinary people living during the first half of the 20th century. They had up to about 30-40 seconds for the body-O2 test, while the medical norm is about 40 seconds.

In order to prove these ideas related to poor health in modern people, let us consider medical evidence related to historical changes in breathing (minute ventilation).

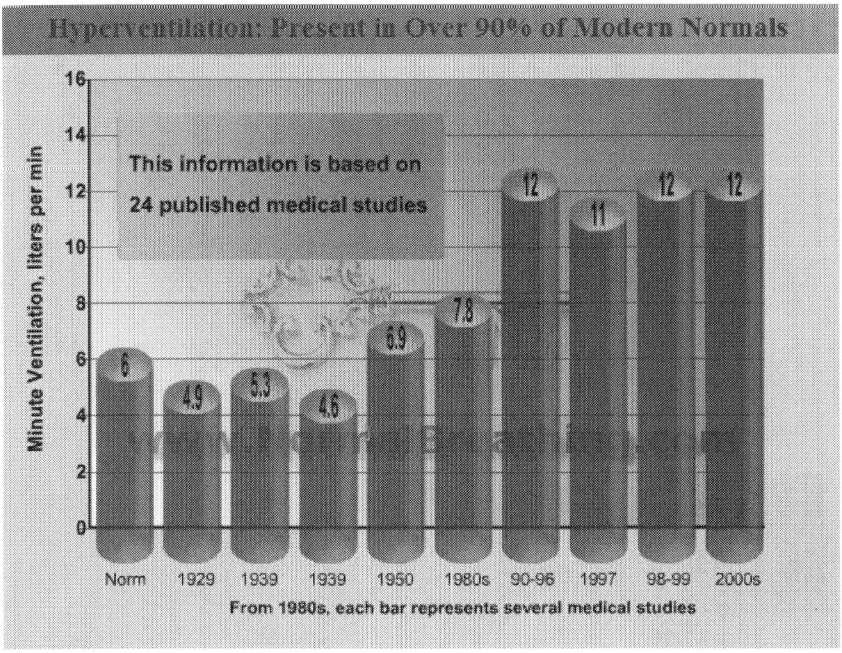

Most people believe that more breathing provides more oxygen for cells, and that CO2 is a toxic gas. However, hundreds of medical studies showed the following results that can be considered as fundamental laws of physiology and respiration.

1. When we breathe more than the medical norm (or hyperventilate), the oxygenation rate of the red blood cells in the lungs remains about the same: 98-99%.

2. Hyperventilation (or breathing more than the medical norm) causes CO2 deficiency (called "hypocapnia") in the lungs, blood and other cells.

3. Since CO2 is the most potent dilator of blood vessels (vasodilator), arterial hypocapnia reduces blood flow to all vital organs of the human body. Hypocapnia also results in the suppressed Bohr effect (or reduced release of oxygen in tissues).

4. As a result, hyperventilation causes reduced perfusion and tissue hypoxia in all vital organs including organs of the digestive system.

5. Tissue hypoxia leads to production of free radicals in cells due to anaerobic cellular respiration. This leads to suppression of the immune system.

Therefore, most contemporary people suffer from reduced blood flow, reduced body oxygenation, and a suppressed immune system. These are the fundamental causes of digestive problems. These causes explain the very low efficacy of common medical treatment (such as antibiotics and surgeries) and alternative health techniques used for digestive problems. All these findings were known to and outlined by the leading Soviet physiologist Dr. Konstantin Pavlovich Buteyko, who invented the Buteyko breathing method to deal with hyperventilation and restore normal breathing and normal body oxygenation.

In relation to GI problems, low CO2 in the arterial blood leads to vasoconstriction and reduced blood flow to the digestive system compromising transfer of oxygen, glucose, digestive enzymes and many other vital nutrients. Low body oxygenation, due to immunosuppression, also allows attachment of pathogens to the mucosal surfaces of the digestive system: in the mouth, throat, stomach, large and small colons, rectum and anus. This leads to formation of biofilms that are very resistant even to medical drugs in people with less than 20 seconds for the body-O2 test. Therefore, on a cell level, the cause of poor digestive health is low body-oxygen levels caused by hyperventilation.

Note that mouth breathing and chest breathing are additional causes of GI problems, since both these factors also reduce body oxygenation. However, both mouth breathing and chest breathing are caused by overbreathing. People with normal breathing naturally (without deliberate effort) have nasal diaphragmatic breathing during sleep and at rest (or for their unconscious breathing).

You can daily eat best supplements, drink canisters of herbal drinks, have hundreds of colonic irrigations, and practice yoga for hours every day, but if your body-oxygen level remains the same, you will likely suffer from the same symptoms and require the same dosage of medication. After applying any treatment that does not change your body O2, your colitis, Candida, gastritis, GERD, or whatever GI problem you have, is likely to come back again (together with accompanying parasites and pathogens) until you increase your body oxygenation to at least 25-30 seconds.

1.4 Body-oxygen test

The DIY body-O2 test is the most fundamental and very accurate health test for more than 99% of people. Clinical experience of over 150 Soviet and Russian MDs showed that this test is possibly the best ever-known health test. How to do this test?

Sit down and rest for 5-7 minutes. Completely relax all your muscles, including the breathing muscles. This relaxation produces a natural spontaneous exhalation (breathing out). Pinch your nose closed at the end of this natural (not deliberate) exhalation and count your breath holding time in seconds. Keep the nose pinched until you experience the first desire to breathe. Practice shows that this first desire appears together with an involuntary push of the diaphragm or swallowing movement in the throat. (Your body warns you, "Enough!") If you release the nose and start breathing at this time, you can resume your usual breathing pattern (in the same way as you were breathing prior to the test).

Do not extend breath holding too long trying to increase the result. You should not gasp for air or open your mouth when you release your nose. The test should be easy and not cause you any stress. This stress-free breath-holding time test should not interfere with your breathing, as shown here:

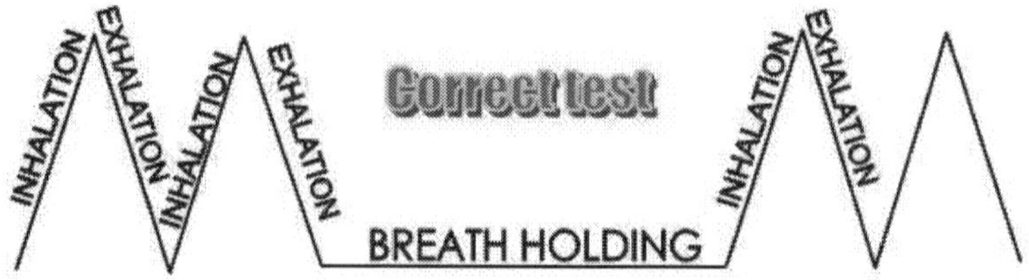

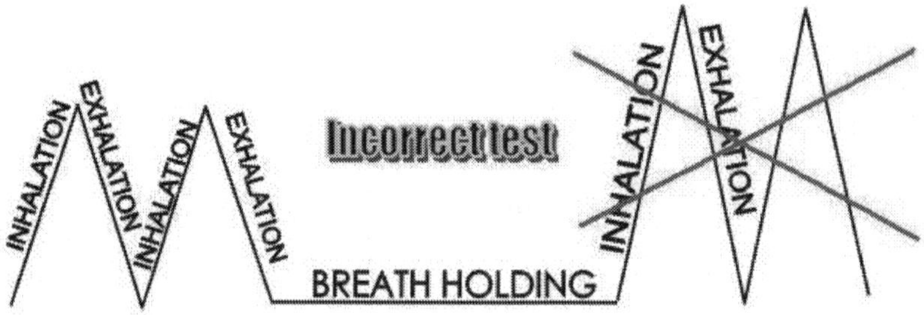

Warning. Some, not all, people with heart disease, migraine headaches, and panic attacks may experience negative symptoms minutes later after this light version of the test. If this happens, they should temporary avoid this test.

This body-O2 test is also called the CP (control pause). This popular abbreviation will be used in the later parts of this book.

CP (control pause) = body-O2 content = breath-holding time after usual exhalation and only until the very first signs of discomfort

What is known about usual CP norms and CPs of sick, normal and healthy people?

"*If a person breath-holds after a normal exhalation, it takes about 40 seconds before breathing commences*" From the textbook "Essentials of exercise physiology", by McArdle W.D., Katch F.I., Katch V.L. (2nd edition), Lippincott, Williams and Wilkins, London 2000, p.252.

Results of Western medical and physiological research studies are summarized in these 2 Tables:

- Body-oxygen test in sick people (13 medical studies; less than 20 seconds)

Condition	Number of subjects	Body Oxygen or Control Pause, s	Reference
Hypertension	95	12 s	Ayman et al, 1939
Neurocirculatory asthenia	54	16 s	Friedman, 1945
Anxiety states	62	20 s	Mirsky et al, 1946
Class 1 heart patients	16	16 s	Kohn & Cutcher, 1970
Class 2-3 heart patients	53	13 s	Kohn & Cutcher, 1970
Pulmonary emphysema	3	8 s	Kohn & Cutcher, 1970
Functional heart disease	13	5 s	Kohn & Cutcher, 1970
Asymptomatic asthmatics	7	20 s	Davidson et al, 1974
Asthmatics with symptoms	13	11 s	Perez-Padilla et al, 1989
Panic attack	14	11 s	Zandbergen et al, 1992
Anxiety disorders	14	16 s	Zandbergen et al, 1992
Outpatients	25	17 s	Gay et al, 1994
Inpatients	25	10 s	Gay et al, 1994
COPD and congenital heart failure	7	8 s	Gay et al, 1994
12 heavy smokers	12	8 s	Gay et al, 1994
Panic disorder	23	16 s	Asmudson & Stein, 1994
Obstructive sleep apnea syndrome	30	20 s	Taskar et al, 1995
Successful lung transplantation	9	23 s	Flume et al, 1996
Successful heart transplantation	8	28 s	Flume et al, 1996
Outpatients with COPD	87	8 s	Marks et al, 1997
Asthma	55	14 s	Nannini et al, 2007

- Body-oxygen test in healthy people (24 references; about 20-30 seconds now; about 40-50 seconds 80-100 years ago)

Types of people investigated	Number of subjects	**Control Pause, s**	References
US aviators	319	**41 s**	Schneider, 1919
Fit instructors	22	**46 s**	Flack, 1920
Home defense pilots	24	**49 s**	Flack, 1920
British candidates	23	**47 s**	Flack, 1920
US candidates	7	**45 s**	Flack, 1920
Delivery pilots	27	**39 s**	Flack, 1920
Pilots trained for scouts	15	**42 s**	Flack, 1920
Min requir. for flying		**34 s**	Flack, 1920
Normal subjects	20	**39 s**	Schneider, 1930
Normal subjects	30	**23 s**	Friedman, 1945
Normal subjects	7	**44 s**	Ferris et al, 1946
Normal subjects	22	**33 s**	Mirsky et al, 1946
Aviation students	48	**36 s**	Karpovich, 1947
Normal subjects	80	**28 s**	Rodbard, 1947
Normal subjects	3	**41 s**	Stroud, 1959
Normal subjects	16	**16 s**	Kohn & Cutcher, 1970

Normal subjects	6	28 s	Davidson et al, 1974
Normal subjects	16	22 s	Stanley et al, 1975
Normal subjects	7	29 s	Gross et al, 1976
Normal subjects	6	36 s	Bartlett, 1977
Normal subjects	9	33 s	Mukhtar et al, 1986
Normal subjects	20	36 s	Morrissey et al, 1987
Normal subjects	14	25 s	Zandbergen et al, 1992
Normal subjects	26	21 s	Asmudson & Stein, 1994
Normal subjects	30	36 s	Taskar et al, 1995
Normal subjects	76	25 s	McNally & Eke, 1996
Normal subjects	8	32 s	Sasse et al, 1996
Normal subjects	10	38 s	Flume et al, 1996
Normal subjects	31	29 s	Marks et al, 1997
Normal males	36	29 s	Joshi et al, 1998
Normal females	33	23 s	Joshi et al, 1998
Healthy subjects	20	38 s	Morooka et al, 2000
Normal subjects	6	30 s	Bosco et al, 2004
Normal subjects	19	30 s	Mitrouska et al, 2007
Healthy subjects	14	34 s	Andersson et al, 2009

Doctor Buteyko and his medical colleagues (about 150 doctors) tested more than two hundred thousand Soviet and Russian patients and found that the following relationships generally hold true for the body-oxygen test:

1-10 s - severely sick, critically and terminally ill patients, often hospitalized

10-20 s - sick patients with numerous complaints and, often, on daily medication

20-30 s - people with average health and usually without serious chronic health problems

40-60 s - very good health

Over 60 s - ideal health, when many modern diseases are virtually impossible.

How does the body-oxygen test relate to your automatic breathing?

Medical evidence suggests that sick people are heavy breathers (you can find these research studies on the Homepage of NormalBreathing.com). Heavier breathing leads to reduced results for this body-oxygen test:

- If you have about 40 seconds for the body-oxygen test, you have normal breathing (with about 5-7 L/min for minute ventilation at rest).

- If your CP is 20 s, you breathe for 2 people or twice more than the medical norm.

- If you have 10 s of oxygen in the body or less, you breathe for at least 4 people.

Hence, if you learn how to breathe slower and less (in regard to your automatic or unconscious breathing), you will naturally increase your body-oxygen levels. It is very difficult, and in many cases nearly impossible, to improve or solve digestive problems without increased body oxygenation.

1.5 Restoration of digestive health: the main goals

Nearly all people with serious digestive problems have less than 20 seconds for the body-oxygen test.

Their digestive problems would be less severe, when they achieve more than 20 seconds for body O2 and maintain the CP at this level 24/7. This is a crucial initial step to achieve significant improvements in GI health. Here is a Chart that describes the main requirements and expected effects.

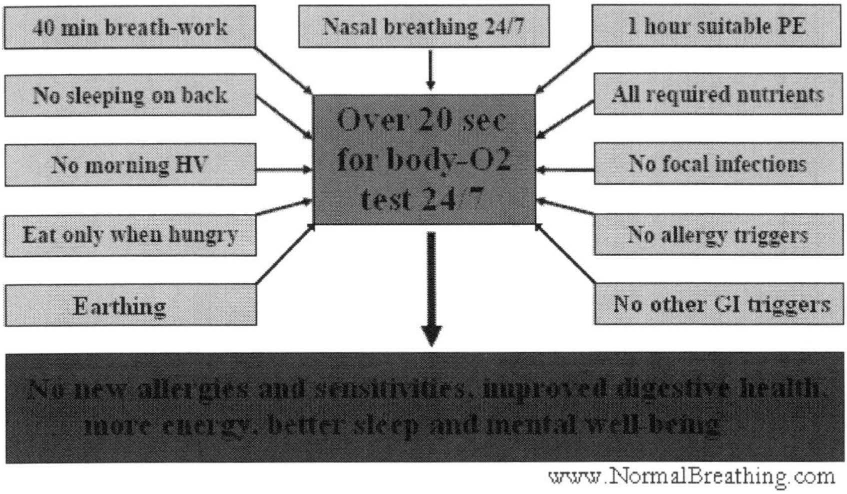

Explanations and notes for this Chart.

A 40 min breath-work program can include 2 breathing sessions each 20 min long, or 3 sessions about 13-14 min long, or 4 sessions at 10 min each. People with some GI problems need to follow special guidelines in relation to breathing exercises.

Among other fundamental steps are **Prevention of breathing through the mouth** and **Prevention of sleeping on one's back**. There are 2 special manuals that can be used, if relevant: the Manual "How to prevent sleeping on one's back" and the Manual "How to maintain nasal breathing 24/7". They are both provided on the main site (NormalBreathing.com).

No morning HV means no morning hyperventilation (i.e., the CP drop throughout the night should be no more than 5 seconds, preferably less than 3 s). You have to solve all sleep-related problems that cause your overnight CP drop.

1 hour suitable PE means 1 hour of total Physical Exercise every day with strictly nasal breathing (in and out) all the time. Usually, less than 20 seconds for the current CP indicates feeling tired and an inability to do running, jogging, or any other rigorous exercise with strictly nasal breathing. However, for most people with GI problems and less than 20 s CP, walking with nose breathing is possible. Moreover, with further CP increase, students feel empowered and surprised by energy and skills previously hidden in their sick bodies.

All required nutrients are discussed later in this book. The most common deficiencies include fish oil, calcium, magnesium, zinc, and protein. Some other nutritional deficiencies can also slow down or even halt breathing retraining. Mild cortisol deficiency and existing GI inflammation can also be corrected using a special program related to Earthing and described in this book.

"**Eat only when hungry**" is the central common sense rule developed by Dr. Buteyko in relation to meals. This rule is particularly important for people with GI problems. It also means that you should stop eating at the first sign of satiety.

No focal infections requires your analysis of certain health conditions that can not be solved using breathing retraining. Breathing retraining is successful against heart disease, asthma, diabetes and even cancer. However, if you have large intestinal parasites (worms), depending on the toxic load, your current CP will be restricted to about 20-35 seconds. The focal infections are able to slow down your GI recovery (for low CP numbers) or even prevent it entirely (when you achieve about 20-35 s CP). There is a separate chapter in this book devoted to focal infections. Focal infections include:

1. Large intestinal parasites (roundworms, flatworms, hookworms, liver flukes, etc.)

2. Dental cavities (caries or pathogenic anaerobes in teeth)

3. Dead tonsils (degenerated tonsils that do not have blood supply and harbor pathogenic bacteria)

4. Feet mycosis (or athlete's foot).

Sometimes, the presence of root canals or mercury amalgams can become the main issue that requires attention (i.e., removal) for higher CP and better health.

No allergy triggers and **No other GI triggers** involve avoidance of any triggers of your allergic reactions and flare-ups. These triggers can include:

- air-born dust mites, cat and dog proteins, mold, pollen, paper ink, cigarette and tobacco smoke (including secondhand smoke), toxic air born chemicals, pollutants, and fumes

- digested gluten products, dairy products, peanuts, tomatoes, and many other foods and substances

- tap water or other consumed liquids with chemical triggers that are present in them

- substances and objects that can produce an allergic response due to skin contact (synthetic clothes, tiny residues of detergents on fabrics, paints, metals, plastics, etc.)

- electromagnetic and other penetrating radiation

- mechanical pressure on abdominal organs due to bending, body twisting, and so on.

These and other examples are considered below.

Regular allergic inflammatory response exhausts cortisol reserves, promotes pathogens in the gut, and suppresses the immune system, making breathing normalization very difficult or even impossible.

Earthing (electrical grounding of the human body) is considered in more detail below.

The main next target: over 30-35 s CP

With over 30 seconds the immune system starts to deal with pathogens and biofilms, dramatically improving the GI symptoms described above. Many GI problems gradually disappear if the person maintains over 30 s CP 24/7.

However, complete elimination of inflammation and restoration of structural integrity of the gut for virtually all GI problems can be achieved with about 35-40 seconds for body O2 24/7.

The next practical observation is that digestive flare-ups cause a variety of problems that lead to reduced body O2 with usually less than 25 s for the body-O2 test. It follows from this observation that getting higher body-O2 numbers requires **avoidance of triggers and allergic reactions** that causes flare-ups. In other words, one cannot normalize breathing, body O2 and health without addressing his or her GI issues.

When teaching breathing retraining to hundreds of students, it was noticed that, for many people, restoration of digestive health (with no soiling effect) is a "side effect" of breathing normalization. They gradually see disappearance of main symptoms and greatly improved or completely normalized digestive health.

However, an increasing number of breathing students worldwide experience serious digestive problems that can not be solved using the standard program of breathing retraining due to negative effects of numerous triggers that cause digestive flare-ups. Such people get stuck at about 20-25 seconds for the body-oxygen test for many months or even years.

Digestive exacerbations or flare-ups create numerous negative effects:

- advance of pathogens and increased toxic load

- formation of GI biofilms in the small intestine

- reduced absorption of nutrients

- worsened inflammation in the gut

- reduced cortisol reserves and general stress

- worsened hormonal profile, leading to fatigue, more problems with sleep, and various psychological and emotional problems

- suppression of the immune system

- possible development of multiple allergies due to immunosuppression.

Therefore, the suggested solution to the GI problems is to address 2 factors at the same time:

- increase body-O2 content using known breathing techniques such as the Buteyko method, combined Frolov-Buteyko therapy, or the Amazing DIY breathing device.

- avoid all triggers and modify lifestyle so as to create conditions for health recovery.

1.6 Expected effects of breathing retraining on common GI problems

Listed below are clinical findings of Russian doctors (my experience with my students confirms their observations) about effects of better body oxygenation and breathing exercises on common GI problems.

• **Chronic gastritis**
- Immediate decrease and, later, complete elimination of pain and symptoms due to dyspeptic effects (heartburn, regurgitation, nausea,

etc.).
- Increase in the CP is accompanied by normalization of colonic tone, phasic contractility of the GI tract, perfusion, metabolic processes in the mucosal surface of the esophagus and stomach, causing accelerated healing of erosions and ulcers, together with regeneration of the mucosal surface of the stomach.
- When the student achieves 35 s for the morning CP and maintains this level for more than 2 weeks, normalization of the immune profile leads to eradication of Helicobacter Pylori.
- Prevention of complications due to chronic gastritis, and complete clinical remission for many years.
- Significant improvements in the quality of life.

• **Chronic non-ulcerative colitis**
- Immediate decrease and, later, complete elimination of pain and symptoms due to dyspeptic effects (bloating and rumbling in the belly, regurgitation, nausea, inconsistencies in bowel habits, etc.).
- Increase in the CP is accompanied by normalization of colonic tone, phasic contractility of the GI tract, perfusion, and metabolic processes in the mucosal surface, leading to its regeneration.
- When the student achieves 40 s CP or more and maintains this level for more than 2 weeks, normalization of the immune profile leads to normalization of the GI flora with elimination of pathogenic bacteria and inflammation in the lining of the large intestine.
- Prevention of complications.
- Complete clinical remission for many years (cure).
- Significant improvements in the quality of life.

• **Chronic pancreatitis**
- Immediate decrease and, later, complete elimination of pain and symptoms due to dyspeptic effects (bloating and rumbling in the belly, regurgitation, nausea, vomiting, alternating bowel habits, etc.).
- Increase in the CP is accompanied by normalized colonic tone, phasic contractility of the GI tract and recovered internal secretion.
- Prevention of complications (diabetes mellitus, pancreonecrosis, secondary diseases of the biliary tract, etc.).
- Complete clinical remission for many years (cure).
- Significant improvements in the quality of life.

• **Chronic cholecystitis**
- Immediate decrease and, later, complete elimination of pain and symptoms due to dyspeptic effects (bloating and rumbling in the belly, regurgitation, nausea, vomiting, alternating bowel habits, etc.).
- Increase in the CP is accompanied by normalization of colonic tone, phasic
contractility of the GI tract, perfusion, metabolism in the lining of the intestine, tone of the bile-conducting organs and elimination of inflammatory processes in the bile-conducting system.
- When the student achieves 35 s morning CP and maintains this level for more than 2 weeks, normalization of the immune profile leads to normalization of the GI flora, disappearance of pathogenic bacteria and elimination of inflammation in the biliary tract.
- Prevention of complications.
- Inhibition of formation of stones in the gallbladder.
- Complete clinical remission for many years (cure).
- Normalization of the emotional life of the students and significant improvement in the quality of life.

• **Gastro-esophageal reflux (GERD)**
- Immediate decrease and, later, complete elimination of pain and symptoms due to dyspeptic effects (heartburn and regurgitation).
- Increase in the CP is accompanied by improved perfusion and normalization of the metabolic processes in the mucosal surface of the esophagus and stomach, with accelerated healing of erosions and ulcers.
- When the student achieves 35 s morning CP and maintains this level for more than 2 weeks, normalization of the immune profile leads to normalization of the GI flora, disappearance of pathogenic bacteria and elimination of inflammation in the esophagus and stomach.
- Prevention of recurring appearances of erosions and ulcers.
- Normalization of the emotional life and significant improvement in the quality of life.

From these typical results, one can infer the similar expected effects for many other GI conditions, such as:

- **inflammatory bowel disease (Crohn's disease and ulcerative colitis)**

- **irritable bowel syndrome**

- **diverticulitis**

- **dyspepsia.**

If an average breathing student with, for example, asthma or hypertension, requires a certain amount of work in order to achieve a certain CP level and corresponding health recovery (with no symptoms are present, and no medication are required), then a student with additional digestive problems often requires at least 2-5 times more effort in order to achieve the same result. This relates to dietary changes, lifestyle changes, breathing exercises, and some other adjustments. It also takes much more effort for a breathing practitioner to restore the health of a student who, in additional to his or her low CP, has serious digestive problems.

A small number of students with GI problems are able to progress smoothly to higher morning CPs (about 30-35 seconds), and their digestive problems cause only a minimum impact on their health recovery. Many breathing-retraining students are slowed down (up to 2 times or more) since they need to learn from mistakes they make. In more serious cases, some breathing students get stuck for months or years (usually with about 15-25 s for the morning CP) due to problems with identifying and addressing all hidden GI factors that prevent their CP growth.

Obviously, our goal is to pinpoint all these adverse factors and empower the person with practical tools to restore their digestive system to its original state as it was designed by Nature.

2. Common triggers of digestive problems

2.1 Allergies

If a person is exposed to any allergic trigger every day and if this trigger creates inflammation in the GI tract, then this person will very likely have less than 30 seconds for the morning CP (most likely less than 25 seconds). An allergic reaction works similar to a focal infection. The final results are: generation of free radicals, advance of pathogens, reduced cortisol reserves, suppression of the immune system, heavier breathing, a lower CP, increased heart rate, and many others.

While there are many allergy tests, one of the best choices is allergy skin prick testing.

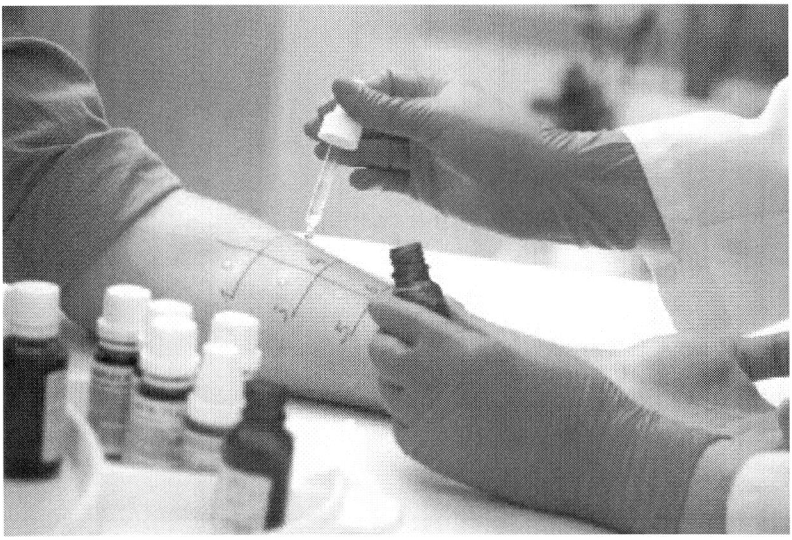

A microscopic amount of an allergen is introduced to a patient's skin, usually with a needle or pin, containing a small amount of the allergen. It is also called a “scratch test”. A single test can include up to 30-40 different substances to be injected under the skin.

After injection of a solution of food or other substance, there are several minutes of waiting time. In cases of allergic reaction, the area around the pricked place becomes swollen and inflamed. The diameter of the inflamed area (which is visible as an inflamed and swollen dome-shaped area) reflects the degree of the reaction. Usually this inflamed area is from 1 to 5 mm in size. It is assumed that the same effects (inflammation and swelling) take place in the GI tract.

Medical professionals are not yet aware about the finding that the results for this prick test, as for any inflammatory reaction, depend on the electrical voltage of the person or presence of grounding (Earthing). When the body is grounded (or electrically connected to the Earth), many allergic reactions do not take place, and even existing inflammation is dramatically reduced. (Surgeons do know about importance of grounding, and all major surgeries are done on grounded patients.)

That means that an insulated person can be positively tested for some food allergy to, for example, oranges or tomatoes. This person can indeed be allergic to oranges or tomatoes but only when he or she is insulated from the Earth and has a positive body charge. It is possible that in conditions of grounding (or while having the same negative voltage as the Earth), this person can safely eat oranges or tomatoes.

Medical professionals also use blood tests for allergies. These tests are more expensive, limited to only one substance (per test), and suffer from the same problem related to the effects of grounding.

Some alternative health practitioners use muscular kinesiology and muscle testing to find allergies. These tests are even less reliable due to additional factors related to unconscious beliefs and psychological denial.

Note that if you have serious digestive problems and have been complaining about these problems to your health care provider for some months, it is very likely that your doctor will either suggest or agree with your request to conduct an allergy prick test. This test is valuable and provides you with practical knowledge related to your immune reactions.

Most common food allergies

There are no exact numbers, but approximate results provided by medical professionals suggest the following. In conditions of electrical insulation, from 50% up to 90% of all severe allergic reactions to foods are caused by:

- *milk*

- *wheat*

- *eggs*

- *peanuts*

- *tree nuts*

- *soy*

- *fish*

- *shellfish.*

Most common allergy triggers

There are other allergy triggers that usually affect the respiratory system or skin. Nearly any of these allergens can cause serious GI distress, especially in conditions of electrical insulation:

- *pollens*

- *animal hair*

- *dust mites and dust mite droppings*

- *insect bites*

- *mold*

- *latex*

- *medical drugs*

- *perfume*

- *secondhand smoke*

- *proteins from feces of cockroaches.*

Usually these allergy triggers affect the respiratory system and/or may cause symptoms of hay fever. However, even though this may look unusual, there are thousands of people who can get GI flare-up and inflammation due to dust mites, perfumes and other triggers.

There are also individuals who experience serious GI exacerbations due to their exposure to, for example, ordinary laundry detergents used to wash their clothes that they wears 24/7. These people can experience constant (hidden) allergic reactions and suffer from digestive problems for years. Other factors may look like triggers. In reality, they may play only a secondary role.

For a person who spends most of his time indoors, chemicals that are used to wash floors or dishes can be triggers. Here are again we have a situation with a hidden, constantly present trigger.

When electrically insulated people wear synthetic fabrics on their skin, these fabrics extract electrons and dramatically increase body voltage to hundreds or even t

housands of volts (creating a positive charge) due to triboelectricity. This positive electrical potential dramatically worsens the inflammatory response.

Note that grounding (or Earthing) is a very new health area. Electrons are able to act as antioxidants to eliminate the destructive effects of reactive-oxygen and reactive-nitrogen species on healthy cells. However, it is possible, that the immune reaction itself (or the chain of multiple events that is involved in the immune response) also depends on grounding.

Therefore, it is smart to get grounded, ideally, nearly all the time, or, at least, when you expect possible allergic triggers or have meals and while you digest them.

If you identified an allergy trigger, you need to follow the most important rule related to your GI recovery:

Rule # 1. Any allergy trigger that causes digestive problems or flare-ups should be avoided.

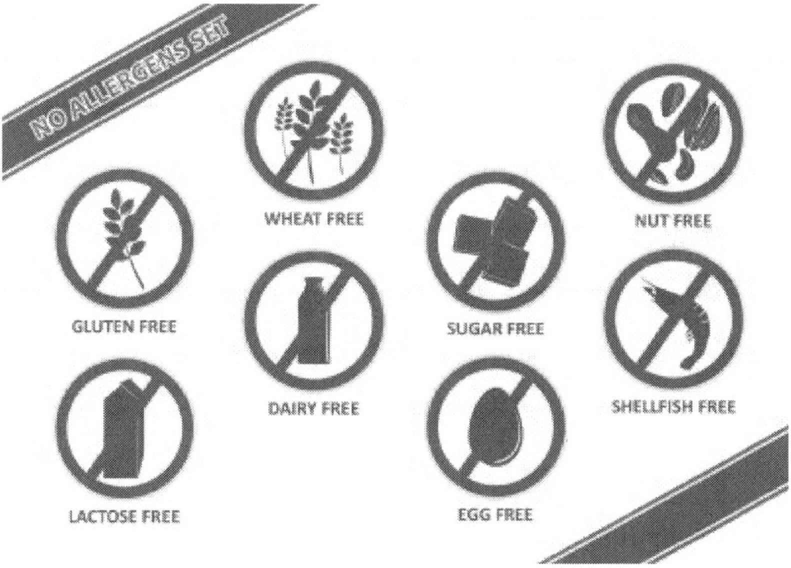

2.2 Chemical triggers present in food and water

Depending on the location and types of existing damage in the GI tract, various chemicals and substances can irritate the inflamed mucosal lining and villi. The effects of irritating chemicals are easier to consider using examples.

Example 1. Raw garlic, raw onions, and other spices

If a person with gastritis eats raw garlic, he or she may notice much more burping some 1-3 hours after the meal. This gas is due to powerful chemicals present in raw garlic. For people with healthy guts, raw garlic is an excellent food. In fact, it is one of the best foods to suppress and destroy Candida yeast infection, and many other parasites often residing in the GI tract. However, the presence of damage and existing inflammation makes mucosal surfaces too weak to resist the strong chemical effects of raw garlic, which destroys mucosal cells in the stomach (and inflamed villi in the small intestine), causing more inflammation, possible thirst (due to swelling of the stomach and colon), and worsened body-O2 content and health.

The same effect can take place in people with damaged GI organs due to eating onions and many other spices, such as black pepper, hot chili pepper, cloves, ginger, and so forth.

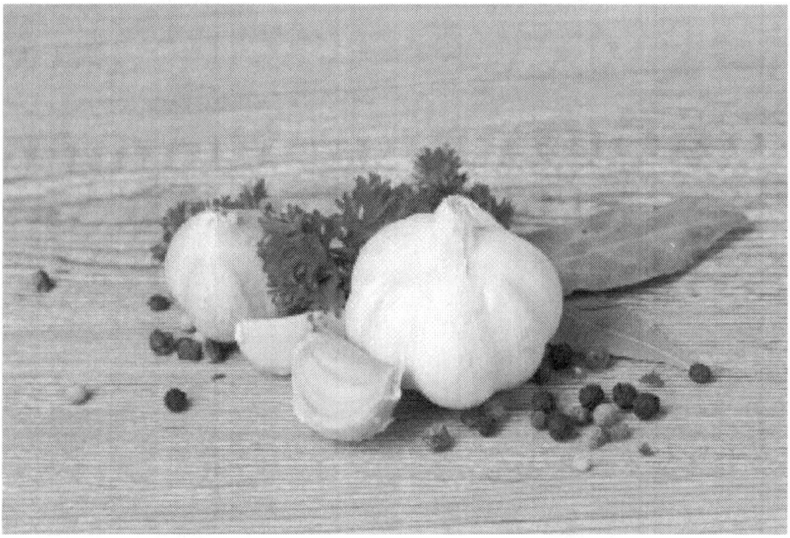

However, when garlic and onions are cooked, the same person with gastritis may not experience any adverse symptoms. Even in cooked form (when enzymes and some other useful chemicals are destroyed due to high temperatures), onions and garlic are still able to fight pathogens in the gut since these foods provide inulin, a type of fiber that is not digested, but becomes food for probiotics or beneficial bacteria that should dominate the healthy gut. Note that some other spices (such as ginger or black pepper) create GI distress even after very long cooking.

Someone else, who has IBS, colitis or Crohn's disease, can also experience the same negative effects of raw garlic or raw onions. The main negative symptoms are likely to appear about 1-4 hours later after the meal.

Example 2. Oranges and other citrus fruits

Here is another example of a chemical trigger. When a person with an irritable bowel syndrome (or Crohn's disease) eats oranges, he or she may notice some adverse effects about 2-4 hours later. These effects can include thirst, flatulence, sleepiness, nausea, mental fog, and some others.

Oranges can be an allergy trigger for the immune system. At the same time, there are other chemicals that are present in oranges that may not cause any allergic reaction, but produce chemical damage to the inflamed lining of the GI tract. What are these chemicals?

When the small intestine is inflamed, acids are able to damage its villi. This relates to citric acid and ascorbic (vitamin C) acid present in oranges and other citrus fruits. Both these acids are generally beneficial for our health. Ascorbic acid is even known as an essential nutrient. However, the inflamed areas of the gut are not able to defend themselves from any of these acids. Even 10 or 50 mg of vitamin C (50 mg is a daily RDA dose) can be sufficient to trigger a digestive flare-up with negative symptoms.

Note that the prick test for oranges and other citrus fruits can be negative (with no allergy triggers). However, any time when citrus fruits are consumed, there can be a negative reaction. Obviously, if a person with such an adverse reaction consumes citrus fruits every day, he or she will not be able to restore the gut.

There is an additional negative factor in most citrus fruits: fructose. People with digestive problems often have Candida Albicans residing in their duodenum (the first part of the small intestine). Candida yeast consumes simple sugars (like those present in nearly all fruits) causing sleepiness, nausea, mood swings and mental fog. When the CP is less than 10 s, Candida can become systemic due to inability of the immune system to resist pathogens even in the blood.

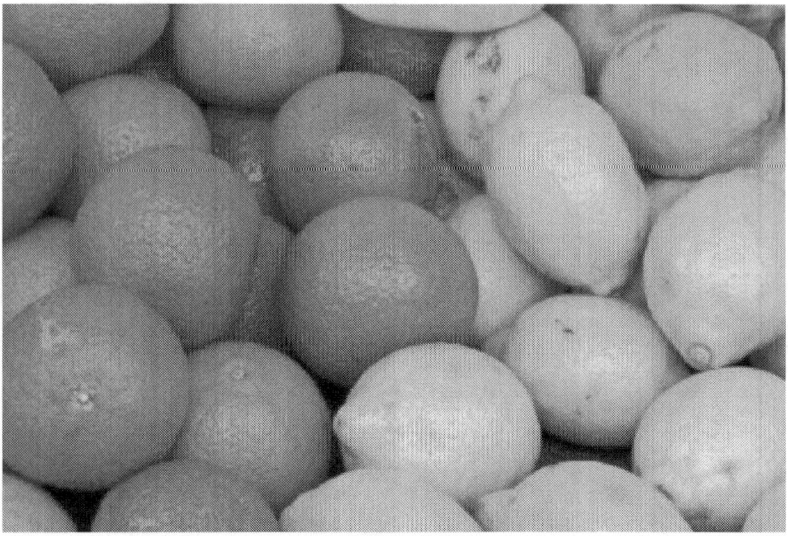

Among all citrus fruits, lemons and limes are safest in relation to Candida, but, as explained above, even lemons and limes can cause adverse effects due to their acids. (The effects of acids can be neutralized with baking soda as we are going to consider below.)

Example 3. Essential oils

Another large group of obnoxious chemicals (but only when the structural integrity of the gut is compromised) includes essential oils.

Not all people with digestive problems are sensitive to essential oils. However, in many cases, the problem is that tiny amounts of essential oils cause chronic irritation and inflammation, while these minuscule amounts of essential oils can be hidden in, for example, a tooth paste or chewing gum that can are used on a daily basis.

Since most people brush their teeth about 2-3 times every day, just this single procedure (tooth-brushing with a tooth paste that contains essential oils) makes digestive recovery for people with, for example, IBD impossible. Most tooth pastes have peppermint, mint, menthol or some other essential oils.

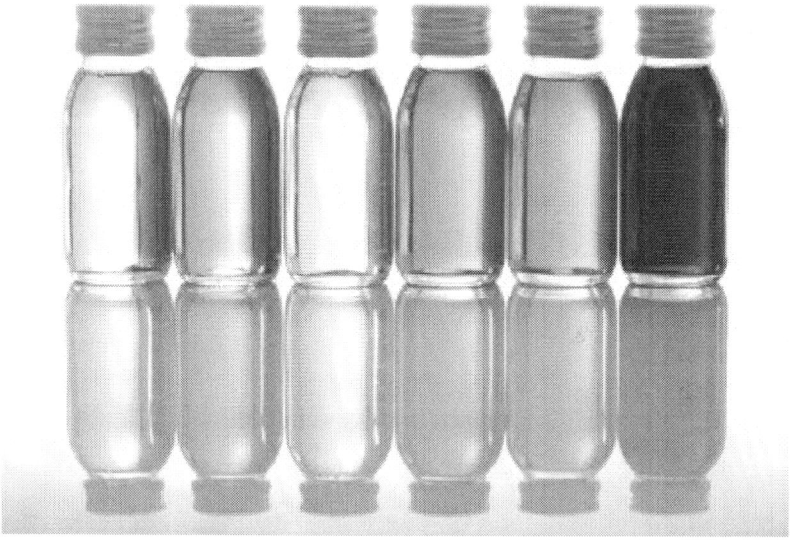

Essential oils are beneficial in diets of people with a normal gut due to the powerful abilities of essential oils to fight pathogens. However, for many people with GI problems, essential oils destroy damaged villi and cause exacerbations of symptoms. If you suspect or are certain about such an adverse reaction to essential oils, get a toothpaste without essential oils such as a toothpaste used for babies or children, and use it until your gut is restored to a better state. Some tooth-whitening pastes are free from essential oils.

The adverse reactions to above-mentioned and some other chemicals are not present in all people with digestive problems. These negative reactions are more common in cases of serious GI problems or severe damage to the stomach or the small or large colon.

If the same person with severe GI problems partially recovers his or her GI health (in an ideal scenario, 1-2 days are enough to achieve the first positive changes), the same person can have much better chances to avoid any negative reactions from the same chemicals due to the improved gut state.

How to reduce or eliminate adverse effects of offensive chemicals

There are 2 useful tips that can either reduce or even completely eliminate the adverse effects of some chemicals.

Tip 1.

Start a meal with some friendly food that can coat the lining of the stomach and the small intestine with a layer that will later prevent the chemical attack of spices and other chemicals. Often, people start their meals with eating spices and other offensive foods first. This causes an immediate chemical attack on the lining of the GI tract. In the suggested scenario, when a person eats some neutral or friendly foods first, the adverse reaction will be either greatly reduced or altogether avoided.

Tip 2.

Acidic substances, such as citric acid and ascorbic acid (vitamin C) can be buffered with baking soda (sodium bicarbonate). You can purchase buffered vitamin C and citric ions in forms of neutral salts. Or you can do it yourself. How to neutralize acids? You will need about a quarter or half of tea spoon of baking soda to neutralize acids in juice from a medium-size lemon. Or you can crush a tablet of vitamin C with a metal spoon in a small cup with water and add about a double volume of baking soda. If you use vitamin C powder (which becomes more common in health food stores and pharmacies), just add it to water, then add about an equal amount of baking soda, and mix them well. The chemical reaction between them (acids and baking soda) lead to formation of carbon dioxide in a form of bubbles or even foam as when you open a bottle or sparkling water or a soda pop.

Note that common or cheap brands of baking soda can be heavily processed and can have aluminum (the same as in table salt). Therefore, you need to find those types of baking soda that claim absence of aluminum ("aluminum-free" or "no aluminum" baking soda). Sometimes a good brand of baking soda can have a label "organic baking soda".

If you take calcium and/or magnesium supplements, it would be a wise step to get magnesium citrate and calcium citrate, which are becoming more common in the USA, Canada, the UK, and other countries. (You can easily find them online as well.) Neutral citric-acid salts usually do not cause any negative reactions even for people with the most severe GI problems.

If we compare the effects of citric and ascorbic acids, ascorbic acid has a stronger negative effect on the inflamed gut. In cases of flare-ups and severe inflammation, even buffered vitamin C (such as sodium ascorbate or calcium ascorbate) can still cause a negative reaction. However, if the same person makes no mistakes and eliminates the biofilms (this may require only 1-2 days), he or she can use buffered ascorbic and citric acids with no adverse effects. Then consumption of buffered vitamin C will be very beneficial to further detoxify the gut.

As we can observe in these examples, a given food or substance can be either beneficial (in cases of good GI health) or destructive (for people with GI problems). The same is true for many activities and lifestyle factors (to be discussed in the next section).

It is also possible to be sensitive to ordinary tap water and conventional foods (or non-organic foods), which usually contain miniscule amounts of various chemicals that can irritate the gut. This topic will be discussed in more detail later in this book.

With the right program of gut restoration, within a few days, the person should be able to re-introduce many previously-destructive substances, chemicals, foods, and activities into his or her diet and lifestyle since they are often useful to speed up the recovery.

2.3 Mechanical triggers

Mechanical pressure on the abdominal area

When some part of the lower gut (located after the stomach) is already inflamed or has an ulcer, or diverticula, or stricture, bending yourself, doing body twisting, and performing other activities that create an additional mechanical pressure on the abdomen and the colon can cause an immediate flare-up (with intensive peristaltic waves leading to swelling of the gut due to additional inflammation, causing possible thirst, flatulence, ear buzzing, and other nearly immediate symptoms). Sometimes, the GI problems can be so severe that a person can have a hard time to tie his or her own shoe laces without creating this GI distress.

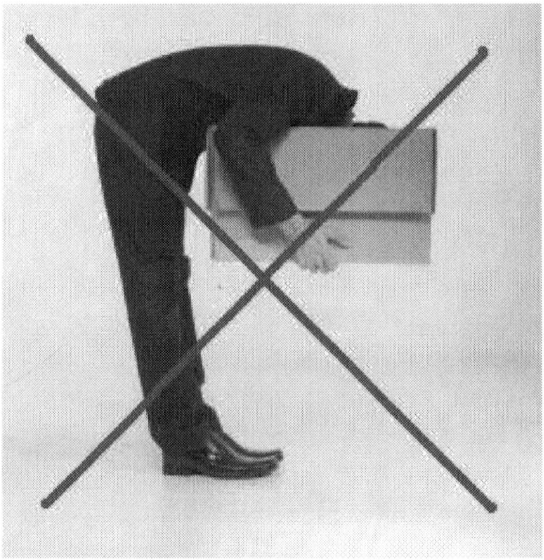

Sleeping in a fetal position can easily cause the same negative effect. In some serious cases, even pressure due to sleeping on a stomach or sides is sufficient to trigger an immediate (usually additional to previous ones) flare-up. With the right behavior this situation can be quickly corrected (within days). More details are provided separately in a section devoted to sleep postures.

Slouching or poor posture is another culprit that is not easy to notice. You need to pay attention to such situations and activities, and possibly be careful with bending forward, side twists and all other activities that can immediately trigger a flare-up.

Some people with digestive problems are able to notice these negative effects. However, sometimes the symptoms are vague and difficult to spot. This often happens in cases with multiple daily triggers that lead to the chronically inflamed and irritable state of the gut.

Pressure on the gut from abdominal muscles

A similar negative effect can take place due to contraction of abdominal muscles. Many activities (such as grating carrots, tooth brushing, physical exercises for training abs, and so forth) can cause an immediate flare-up as well. In some people even scratching some itchy body part causes the same effect.

Therefore, a person with serious GI problems should keep an eye on effects of significant (or repetitive) activities with involvement of the main abdominal muscles: transverse abdominal, the internal obliques, the external obliques, and rectus abdominis.

Shaking of the body and the effects of mechanical vibrations

Other mechanical triggers of flare-ups include those situations that are accompanied by intensive mechanical vibrations of the body as during jumping or running. When one has a duodenal or gastric ulcer, intensive vibrations that are transmitted to internal organs can make the lesion or ulcer open due to its low mechanical strength.

There are similar dangers when structural integrity of other GI organs is compromised due to tumors, diverticula, hernias, and other abnormalities.

Generally, shaking and vibration of the body are beneficial for human health due to positive effects on metabolism, lymphatic drainage, and increased strength of bones and other body parts and tissues. Dr. K. P. Buteyko was among first physiologists who suggested this idea. The body gets healthier and stronger due to its adaptation to mechanical stress. However, when the body is already damaged, mechanical vibrations can have a serious destructive power.

Apart from running and jogging, what are other possible examples with intensive body vibrations? Grating carrots or rigorous mechanical body shaking due to brushing teeth can trigger a flare-up. (Here we can see that tooth-brushing can have 3 independent triggers: essential oils, contraction of abdominal muscles and body vibrations, all of which can trigger a flare-up.)

It is known that falling down or being in car accidents cause more serious problems to people who already have damaged or weak body organs. The negative effects of such accidents are more common in elderly people, who often have worse GI health, structural GI abnormalities and reduced mechanical strength of GI organs.

Running or jumping can cause the lesions of the ulcer to open. The same activities can produce other types of damage to already injured digestive organs. Sometimes, even ordinary walking can lead to adverse symptoms.

In most-severe cases, there are individuals who can not stand up (after sitting) without a flare-up and desire to urinate. Such people need to learn how to stand up slowly in order to strengthen their problematic areas (or weak parts) of the GI system. Application of other methods (such as correct physical exercise, massaging devices, Earthing, and other methods) will quickly (in 1-2 days) help to achieve partial GI recovery. Then the person can do the same activities (e.g., standing up and walking with an ordinary speed but with an empty stomach) without negative effects.

The negative effect of sudden jerks or too-intensive body vibrations, when present in people with ulcers, can be much stronger after meals since presence of the food (or even water) in the stomach makes it much heavier. Therefore, just after meals, even smaller vibrations or jerks can open the lesions of the ulcer. In some cases, such people can easily tolerate strictly vertical vibrations (such as while travelling in a car or train), but have negative reactions to vibrations that involve side-to-side movements.

We can see that in this area (effects of mechanical factors on GI health), there is a wide spectrum of reactions. These bodily reactions also depend on the position of ulcers and other abnormalities.

You need to pay good attention to which types of exercise are ok for you right now and which should be temporary avoided.

2.4 Allergic reactions via skin, air, and EMF fields

While other types of allergies and hypersensitivities are rare, there are still thousands of people who regularly experience digestive flare-ups due to other causes.

For example, if their skin is in contact with synthetic fabrics, especially when they are not grounded, such people will react with diarrhea, burping, bloating, and many other negative GI effects. The effect can be much stronger at low CPs (less than 20 s).

Another type of reaction leading to a digestive exacerbation can take place due to skin contact with fabrics that were washed using ordinary detergents (we considered this example above). In order to avoid such reactions, you can use either hypoallergic, or dermatologically-tested detergents or those detergents that are designed for washing the clothes of babies.

Certain chemicals in air, such as tree pollen, some perfumes, smoke (including secondhand smoke) and other chemicals, can trigger digestive flare-ups or cause a chronic reaction, leading to constant inflammation.

Finally, there are cases when exposure to EMF (electromagnetic fields) produces a nearly-immediate adverse digestive response. This can take place due to wearing a cell phone in a pocket for only for 1-2 minutes or standing for a few seconds next to a working microwave, kettle or electrical oven.

2.5 Negative effects of some breathing exercises

There are 2 types of dangers due to breathing exercises and manipulation of breathing.

A. When solid food is in the stomach

Many breathing students get so obsessed with reduced breathing that they start doing it nearly all the time or whenever they are awake. While this strategy can help to increase the CP and improve one's health for some students, many people get problems when they do RB with solid food in the stomach. With food in the stomach, only people with very strong stomachs and good digestion are able to get benefits from light air hunger and increased CO2 (without any damage). Most people need to avoid any breathing manipulations during and after meals until the stomach is empty.

B. When biofilms are present

Breathing exercises and breath holds can also cause problems even when the stomach has no solid food. An increase in CO2 is a chemical trigger that causes mechanical effects (intensified peristalsis) and enhanced sensitivity of the immune system. Therefore, strong air hunger, long pauses, and large CO2 increases; all these factors can lead to intensive peristaltic waves that can destroy already-inflamed villi. Here is an example:

A person with about 25 s for their current CP starts practicing an intensive breathing session and increases his results for up to 35 or higher numbers for intermediate breath holds while doing Buteyko reduced breathing with strong air hunger. This immediately causes unquenchable thirst and ear buzzing, with bloating and burping appearing later. Even though the final CP after the session is higher, the final heart rate, due to increased inflammation, also gets higher. Within 1 hour after the session, the CP drops to about 20-25 s. Later effects are increased urination, intestinal gas, greasy stool (with increased soiling), cold feet, poor mood, and many others. Why do these effects take place?

Since many people with digestive problems suffer from GI dysbiosis, abnormal GI flora in the gut, and biofilms in the small intestine, this sudden CO_2 and CP increase leads to intensive peristalsis since the body tries to get rid of pathological content in the small and large intestines. This effect of strong peristalsis is generally beneficial: the gut tries to flush out pathogens and their toxins. Such a positive reaction, in the form of diarrhea, takes place, for example, after food poisoning. Higher CO_2 and CPs intensify this effect: you probably noticed that it is much easier to have a bowel movement with breath holds and reduced breathing. (In fact, instead of straining the abdominal muscles, people should do reduced breathing to have an easier bowel movement.)

However, when the mucosal surface of the small intestine is inflamed and covered with biofilms, the damaged villi are weak. Intensive peristaltic waves can easily cause the villi covered with pathogens to be broken and wiped down along the GI tract. All these processes take place beyond the stomach and, as a result, broken villi cannot be digested and used by the body. Instead, these nutrients start to putrefy in the large colon, which, in such cases, is full of pathogens that will "enjoy" proteins and other nutrients from the broken villi in the warm moist conditions of the large colon. This, in turn, will produce toxins in the blood, offensive smell before or during the next bowel movement, increased soiling, marks on the toilet, and other negative effects.

Such a severe GI reaction due to breathing exercises occurs in students with existing GI damage due to colitis, Crohn's disease, IBS (irritable bowel syndrome), and some other conditions with biofilms on the lining of the small intestine.

Sometimes, the gut is so damaged that even a light reduced breathing with food in the stomach or the CP test on an empty stomach can cause a GI exacerbation.

The tricky part here is that such flare-ups are easy to induce. The body readily "accepts" reduced breathing and makes a quick transition (in 1-2 minutes) to higher CO2 with a large temporary CP increase. This is particularly easy to achieve with maximum breath holds or maximum pauses.

In contrast, when biofilms are absent, and the same (or other) person practices reduced breathing, it takes much more effort to slow down breathing due to normal (inherent) resistance of the breathing center to higher CO2. As a result, one may spend 10-12 minutes on breathing exercises before the breathing center yields to higher CO2.

How to prevent practicing reduced breathing with food in the stomach? One of the suggested solutions for such people is to practice humming through the nose immediately after meals while food is in the stomach.

Another part of the same problem is that some Western Buteyko practitioners declare to their students that these adverse symptoms (with intestinal gas, bloating, diarrhea, soiling and other effects) are signs of a "body cleanse" or "body detoxification" due to higher CPs caused by breathing exercises, even though this reaction can be present for many months. As a result, their breathing students continue the same intensive breathing sessions that destroy their new villi and cause inflammation every day. The main effect of such intensive breathing exercises is the destruction of the GI tract, leading to a cascade of negative events involving worsened inflammation, increased urination, flatulence, foul odor, cortisol deficiency, fatigue, poor sleep, mood swings and many other negative effects. Most of all, the morning CP remains at about 20-25 s.

2.6 Synergetic effect of GI triggers

Any 2 or more GI triggers, when they occur at the same time, produce disproportionally stronger negative effects in comparison with a simple sum of their effects. In other words, a little bit of one adverse factor and a little bit of another adverse factor together can cause an avalanche in the gut.

When the same person, just a few days later, partially recovered his or her gut, the same triggers have much less power (but they still can reduce the gut to its initial damaged state). Why do existing GI problems make people more sensitive to other triggers?

This is because the presence of biofilms on the mucosal surface of the gut is a large initial factor, while additional triggers are greatly amplified due to a presence of biofilms. This also explains why digestive problems can often last for years, and why they require a comprehensive program of diet and lifestyle changes.

2.7 Sequences of negative symptoms for digestive flare-ups

When a person has heartburn, this symptom of acid reflux (and sometimes acid taste in the mouth) is obvious. Similarly, burping due to gastritis is another easily noticeable sign. Blood on a toilet paper is also easy to notice. These symptoms are usually accompanied by many others, such as soiling, coating on the tongue, flatulence, and offensive smell.

However, the symptoms of a flare-up in the duodenum or the small intestine, due to duodenal ulcers, Crohn's disease, or IBS, can often be vaguer and can remain unnoticed for many hours after the meal. These symptoms often have a typical sequence that can slightly vary from person to person.

When the small intestine is involved, one of the common sequences, after a flare-up, is the following. The person eats a wrong food or does something that causes problems for the small intestine (e.g., rigorous tooth brushing with essential oils). The very first sign can be ear buzzing due to mechanical or chemical damage to the gut. This noise is likely coming from the enteric nervous system that orchestrates the work of the GI system. This is the initial stage of a flare-up, when many villi in the small intestine get destroyed. In order to protect the lining of the gut from further damage, neighboring cells swell and get inflamed (in cases of ungrounded people; electrical grounding minimizes these negative effects on surrounding healthy tissues). Damaged tissues draw a large amount of water to the small intestine. As a result, the next symptoms are heaviness in the abdominal area, moist nose (or moister nose than it was before), and unquenchable thirst: an unpleasant sensation of dryness on lips (similar to thirst) that cannot be reduced even by drinking 1 or 2 liters of water.

There are also delayed effects for this typical flare-up. Once villi are inflamed and partially destroyed (and some of them can be wiped down the gut with this meal or the next one), putrefaction of villi in the colon occurs. In other words, your tissues start to rot inside yourself. This process of their disintegration by pathological bacteria usually takes many hours. The conditions in the gut are ideal for putrefaction: warm temperature, high humidity, and large concentrations of different pathogens that will be happy to digest your proteins, lipids, blood nutrients, and other substances from broken villi by converting them into toxins to poison the body and drive the body O2 and health down 24/7.

Note that proteins are digested mainly in the stomach. Bacteria and other pathogens that we eat with food also need to go through the stomach (where they get either weakened or killed). However, decay of villi takes place beyond the stomach. Therefore, the body is defenseless against this effect. The only partial solution of the body, for this hard challenge, is to expel the polluted content of the large intestine with bowel movements.

Inflammation and swelling of the small colon presses on the walls of the urinary bladder, creating an urge to urinate even when one has only 100-200 ml of urine in the bladder. Therefore, the next (measurable) symptom is increased frequency of urination and reduced volume of urine per one toilet trip. For many people, the amount of urine that can be stored in the urinary bladder is a very sensitive parameter that accurately reflects their current GI health.

Putrefaction of own tissues in the colon leads to another set of symptoms that appear hours later. These later or delayed symptoms usually include cold feet, bloating, flatulence, intestinal gas, loose and greasy stool (or diarrhea) with foul smell, possible rectal itching, increased soiling, dirty water in the toilet bowl, fatigue, nausea, mental fog or reduced focus and concentration, worse sleep, and many others.

Villi can re-grow with an amazing speed (in about 8-12 hours), but they require about 1-2 days of ideal conditions in order to become mechanically strong and resilient in relation to raw greens, vegetables and other rough foods, as well as various chemicals (as we discussed above).

Our goal is to reveal and adhere to those factors and lifestyle parameters that create conditions for villi to re-grow and mature. In order to discover these ideal conditions (which are very individual), you need to pay close attention or even record all details after each meal and after possible exposure to other situations that can cause such digestive exacerbations.

Note that this Chapter considered most common triggers causing digestive flare-ups. Addressing all these above-discussed triggers can help many, but not all people since there are dozens of other triggers and factors (such as sleep and sleeping positions, water quality, pesticides and herbicides, and so forth). We are going to look at other triggers in more detail later.

2.8 Healthy villi and summary of putrefaction effects

If we imagine that the small intestine is a hollow tube, its surface area will be less than one square meter. This area is greatly increased due to the existence of villi and the convoluted shape of the small colon with numerous folds. The ability of the GI tract to effectively absorb nutrients is based on the existence of normal villi since the total surface area of the small intestine in an adult is over 200 square meters (or more than 2,000 square feet). Therefore, the presence of healthy villi and the convoluted shape of the small colon increase the area for absorption of nutrients more than several hundred times.

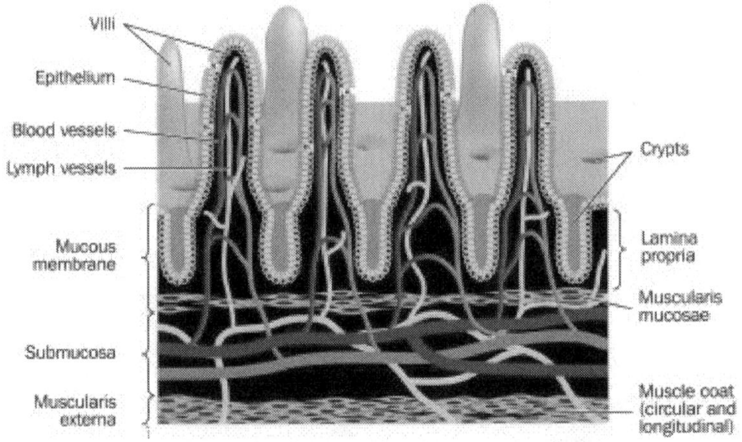

However, in cases of typical GI flare-ups, as in Crohn's disease and colitis, large areas of the small intestine can be wiped out. A typical flare-up causes serious negative effects:

- inability to effectively absorb nutrients

- a need to spend amino acids and resources of the immune system to repair the villi

- a severe GI pollution caused by putrefaction of destroyed villi. (By definition, "putrefaction" is decomposition of organic matter, especially protein, by microorganisms, resulting in the production of foul-smelling matter).

The last effect becomes more apparent if you realize that proteins are mainly digested in the stomach due to low pH and digestive enzymes secreted by the wall of the stomach. Since villi are located below the stomach, their proteins cannot be reused for direct absorption. Instead of being recycled, proteins and amino acids of destroyed villi become food for gut pathogens that generate toxins and other harmful substances.

2.9 Why does the gut react with diarrhea?

A digestive exacerbation or flare-up does not always mean an immediate bowel movement. However, it implies a significant intensification of peristalsis in the small colon. This means that the food is going to travel through the small intestine many times faster than the normal time (a few hours). Obviously, this fast transit time prevents effective absorption of nutrients. Furthermore, these nutrients, instead of building the body, are transformed into harmful substances that are going to poison the body. The question is: what are the causes of this seemingly strange effect?

The GI system reacts with a digestive flare-up when it feels (or calculates) that a possible damage due to normal peristalsis can cause more harm for the body rather than the damage created by putrefaction.

Imagine that you swallowed some sharp object (such as a small porcupine), and this object is not in the small intestine. If the GI system tries to digest this object and moves it back and forth and to the sides in the small intestine, this sharp object can shred the tissues of the small intestine into pieces, and you may die due to severe blood losses. In order to prevent this damage, the GI system rushes this offensive object into the large colon.

A similar effect takes place when the person with IBD eats raw vegetables or nuts. These raw foods can produce significant damage to the lining of the weak and damaged small intestine. Therefore, a digestive exacerbation is a protective mechanism that helps the organism to prevent a more significant damage.

Appearance of chemical irritants, such as spices and essential oils, can also cause large damage if these substances remain in the small intestine for long time. Therefore, the GI system eliminates them rapidly in order to have less destruction.

2.10 Effects of poor digestive health on body O2 and general health

Abnormal digestive flora also creates a serious negative effect on the CP and health of ordinary people. If you already practiced breathing exercises, you know that it requires effort and time even to increase the CP by 3-5 seconds. The body, for some reasons, resists easier breathing and higher O2 content. This effect of resistance can be very strong, but it also can be nearly absent in other people or at other times.

For example, a healthy child can sometimes have up to 50-60 s CP. But the same child can have large CP fluctuations: the CP can drop down to about 10 s. Imagine that this healthy child, whose CP is about 10 s, does the same breathing session (about 12-20 minutes), as you or some other adult. What would be the final CP of this child? It will be about 50-60 s. Why couldn't another adult or you get the same high CP in 12-20 minutes? You may even start with much higher CPs than the child, but your increase would be only about 5 s or slightly more. The child gets better results because the body of the healthy child is clean and has no resistance to easier breathing.

What are the causes of resistance in adults and sick children, who never have high CPs? There are abnormal tissues, toxic chemicals, and numerous pathogens present in different body organs and parts. They all drive the CP down. For example, airway inflammation in a person with asthma is a negative factor that makes breathing heavier and slows down his or her CP progress. When people consume medical drugs, these drugs accumulate in body cells (especially in fat cells) and intensify breathing. Finally, there are various pathogens residing in and on the human body.

The contribution of these pathogens can vary. For people with existing tissue abnormalities (such as airway inflammation in asthmatics), the contribution of abnormal flora in the gut can be small: let say only about 10-20% of the total resistance to CP increase. However, when the same asthmatics starts to avoid triggers of asthma and gets up to 25-30 s CP, then the negative effect of the gut can reach 50% or more.

For people who do not have any physiological pathology (or physical illness), the negative effect of GI flora can account for up to 50-90% of total resistance to their CP increase. Indeed, if they do not have abnormal tissues in the body and did not consume large amounts of drugs, there should be a cause of their inability to increase their CP to very large numbers within one breathing session. The only remaining source of pollution is due to body pathogens, and most pathogens (well over 90%) are usually located in the gut.

Toxic load from pathogens also drives down the morning CP, which is the key measurable factor that reflects our health. Since the putrefaction in the gut takes place 24/7, the toxins from the gut should cause overnight CP drop.

These are also the reasons why no-soiling is an important factor and one of the requirements for breathing students who want to break through 40 s for the morning CP. To get over 40 s MCP is the most difficult challenge in breathing retraining, and even here good digestive health plays a significant role.

3. Symptoms and signs to monitor

After weeks or months of digestive problems, most people have certain patterns related to their digestive symptoms. These patterns can range from very regular to totally erratic. Sometimes, the sufferers are able to pinpoint some or nearly all causes of their problems. In other cases, they have only vague ideas about what is going on in the gut and why they get their specific problems.

3.1 Commonly known symptoms

Many of these symptoms are discussed in books, articles, internet posts, and other sources devoted to GI health. These symptoms include:

- *Bloating*

- *Belching*

- *Flatulence*

- *Diarrhea*

- *Constipation*

- *Fullness*

- *Nausea*

- *Rectal itching*

- *Tongue coating*

- *Thirst.*

Apart from these symptoms, there are many others that often provide even more accurate information about the gut state.

3.2 Frequent-urination log

If you suffer from reduced urinary volume, it is useful to have exact measurements related to timing of trips to the bathroom and exact numbers for the urinary output: e.g., 300 ml, 450 ml, 400 ml, etc. for each trip. (If you prefer cups or some other units of measurement, you can surely use them.)

Recording details in a log will help you to identify triggers of your flare-ups. Males can measure urinary volumes by using a bottle with a large hole, like a Gatorade bottle, and measure the amount of urine and timing of each trip (+-5-10 min) so that to find out the gap between toilet trips. Females may need a basket and a measuring cup.

After some days of measurements, there is no longer any need to collect urine. One can simply count the duration of urination in seconds (with a clock/watch or using mental counting).

The greater the inflammation, the more frequent the urination (the number of trips to a washroom) and the less its volume. In many cases, these numbers are the most indicative measurable parameters for the gut state and conditions you created. As soon as you make a mistake (or have a flare-up), your urinary output becomes smaller. Some of the possible mistakes were discussed above. When you are on the right track, you can naturally keep more urine in the urinary bladder naturall~~y and~~ will have less frequent toilet trips.

For example, during exacerbations, a person may hold only about 150-250 ml (less than 1 cup) and have bathroom trips every 3 hours or even more often (especially in cases of reactive hyperglycemia or high blood glucose). During recovery, the same person may hold up to 700-900 ml and have trips only every 7-10 hours.

3.3 Soiling effect

The degree of soiling and the amount of required toilet paper are easy to monitor. The great thing about the system described in this book is that there is a clear goal in relation to digestive health: to achieve no soiling.

When soiling is present and there are no digestive infections causing diarrhea, it is most likely that the person made a mistake that took place within the time period starting from 2 meals before.

Sometimes, soiling does not mean any serious mistakes, but is caused by a soft diet, or a raw diet, or large amounts of honey.

3.4 Ear buzzing

This symptom is nearly an immediate one. As soon as the small intestine is under stress (with ongoing damage to villi), ear buzzing either appears or becomes more intense.

A modern environment is usually full of noises. As a result, it is often not easy to notice and remember the degree of ear buzzing at each moment of time. Since people with GI problems have ear buzzing for months, they simply stop paying attention to this symptom that becomes hidden in other background noises. You may need to find a quiet place or close your eyes, and listen for 10-15 seconds to hear buzzing or high-pitch noises that are produced within the body.

When the gut starts to repair, ear buzzing can disappear completely. In some people, even during recovery, it can be present in the evenings, after 6 or 9 pm. There are also cases, when during GI recovery, people experience ear buzzing only when they make a transition to a horizontal position for night sleep.

3.5 Unquenchable thirst due to recent GI exacerbation

Unquenchable thirst is a common sign that often reflects the fact that the small intestine has been damaged, became inflamed, and requires more water due to swelling. This can happen due to mechanical damage or other causes. For example, a sudden jerk of the whole body, for a person with damaged GI organs, can make him or her thirsty within 1-2 minutes due to a flare-up. Bending forward or jumping can cause the same nearly immediate effect.

Mechanical damage to the small villi of the small intestine due to poor chewing can also lead to unquenchable thirst. Imagine a person with Crohn's disease or IBD. If this person eats raw vegetables (such as Broccoli, cauliflower, and many others), even while chewing these foods very well, he or she can feel thirst at the time when particles of this food will pass through the inflamed parts of the small intestine.

Similarly, taking unbuffered acidic supplements (such as vitamin C and citric acid) can also cause unquenchable thirst. The same is true for many spices and other irritating substances.

Another possible cause of unquenchable thirst (and GI damage) is too high blood sugar levels. This factor and how to solve problems with hyperglycemia will be discussed below.

3.6 Moist nose

This is another nearly immediate parameter that tells you the story with water turnover in the gut. Flare-ups in the small intestine can result in a very moist noise. During recoveries, it is common for a light crust to form on the nose which makes the nose a little bit itchy since the drying crust pulls the mucosal surfaces of the nose together. The formation of this crust often signifies that biofilms are eliminated and the villi are in a better state.

The formation of a light crust should not be confused with a blocked nose due to infections caused by low CP (less than 20 s). Here, we are considering those situations with a light crust in the nose when one has about 20 s or more for the current CP.

When a person is in good or excellent health, the nose is not too moist and not dry. It is in an intermediate state with little moisture and very little mucus (just enough to do the job).

A moist nose should not be confused with **nasal drip**. People who had serious respiratory or sinus infections in the past and whose nasal passages still harbor remnants of pathogens can experience transitory nasal drip, when they push their CPs up. This can happen at 25-30 s CP, or even sometimes at higher numbers (up to 50-55 s CP). This is an example of a local cleansing reaction that usually lasts only for 2-4 days. It can suddenly appear and suddenly disappear due to higher CP numbers.

3.7 Cold feet

Many people have constantly cold feet due to poor circulation (low arterial CO_2 constricts arteries and arterioles). This symptom often disappears at about 20 s CP (people with hypothyroidism may need higher numbers). However, cold feet are also common among people with digestive problems. Apart from low CP, there is an additional contribution to cold feet due to toxins generated by pathogens located in the gut. As a result, people with GI problems have a tendency to have cold feet even at higher CPs of 20-30 s. In addition, while the breathing of people with digestive problems may remain nearly unchanged (with about 20-25 seconds for the body-oxygen test), their feet become colder or warmer depending on the state of the gut.

This symptom is not an immediate one (it takes time for positive and adverse changes to develop), but cold feet is another useful parameter that makes a person more certain about either exposure to triggers or right actions.

Certain pathogens, such as Blastocystis hominis, cause very cold feet. Blastocystis hominis infections are common in people who have problems digesting fats, usually due to poor liver function.

Candida Albicans and larger parasites (intestinal worms) also contribute to colder feet.

When a person is on his or her road for digestive recovery with increased body-O_2 content, he or she nearly always experiences a pleasant sensation of natural warmness in the feet. There are even cases when recovering people experience heat in their feet, a sensation that they have not had for months or years.

3.8 Mental states

Presence of biofilms in the gut (together with the constantly moist nose, soiling, and other signs of poor GI flora) have a strong effect on mental states of the person. Many GI pathogens generate powerful neurotoxins that have direct adverse effects on the brain and nerve function including concentration, focus, planning and other mental qualities. Poor GI health means confusion, procrastination, excessive anxiety or depression, panic attacks, indecisiveness, and many other negative symptoms.

Such negative mental states can be caused by overbreathing and low body O2 (usually less than 20 seconds). However, nearly all these adverse symptoms are greatly reduced or disappear altogether with higher CPs. In many cases, about 25 s CP is enough to achieve large improvements in the mental area. When biofilms are present, the same 20-25 s CPs do not mean a clear mind and good concentration. The existing GI flora has an independent negative effect on mental well-being. Toxins released by Candida yeast are particularly strong in their mental effects.

Therefore, in addition to physical symptoms, one can monitor his or her mental states. Usually the negative effects in this area relate to the presence of biofilms (the same as with, for example, cold feet). As soon as the biofilms start to disappear, there are improvements.

3.9 Body O2 monitoring

The body-oxygen test is highly sensitive to digestive problems. Mistakes related to digestion cause heavier breathing at rest and reduced body-O2 content. The CP drop is usually at least 5 or more seconds.

Since the ultimate goal of better GI health is to increase body oxygenation, it is clear that CP recording helps to monitor one's GI health. The CP monitoring is particularly useful during the transitory period when one is likely to experience some unusual digestive symptoms and effects.

3.10 Why to record pulse?

Pulse is good to record since it can indicate many problems like GI flare-ups, low calcium, low cortisol, allergy effects, loss of CO_2 sensitivity, and so on. Pulse also reflects the degree of inflammation in the digestive system or other body parts. With higher CP and general progress in digestive health, the pulse gets lower.

If the heart rate of a person with IBD, after Buteyko breathing exercises, increases, this can indicate that the session likely caused GI distress due to too large of a CO_2 increase. In such cases, increased heart rate helps a student to be more certain about the negative effects of incorrect breathing exercises, while reduced heart rate is a sign of correct breathing exercises.

4. Body weight

When humans have less than 20 s CP, it is very common for them to accumulate body fat (due to specific effects of overbreathing on blood sugar control). Most people gain more weight when their CPs become even lower. However, in people with serious GI problems (with weak liver, GI bleeding, cachexia, night sweats, and so on) weight loss is common as well.

The easiest solution to normalize body weight is the same for both cases: as a first step, it is important to increase body oxygenation up to 20 seconds. Then a partial normalization of main physiological functions will help to move one's weight in the right direction. The next step is to get over 30 s CP.

4.1 Effects of breathing exercises on overweight people

When people suffer from chronic overbreathing, most of them are going to accumulate more fat. This happens because chronic overbreathing usually reduces blood glucose levels. Low blood sugar causes low energy, weak muscles, poor mood, grumpiness, abnormal brain function (up to severe migraines) and hunger. As a result, one needs to eat. After meals, blood glucose raises and the symptoms of hypoglycemia are solved, but overbreathing becomes more intense. This leads to formation of a vicious circle where hyperventilation and low body O2 are the key hidden factors that cause weight gain.

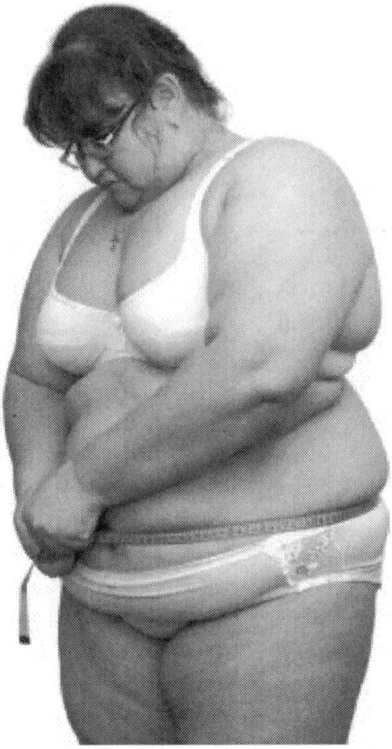

The obvious solution is to slow down breathing. Increased CP means higher blood glucose levels without eating foods. The body starts to use its own reserves.

Therefore, when people are overweight and they increase their body O2, they have much more energy, higher blood sugar levels, and greatly reduced or absent hunger, especially in relation to fats and complex carbohydrates. As a result, it is easy and natural to lose weight with those breathing exercises and lifestyle changes that increase body oxygenation.

I have seen this effect in hundreds of breathing students. When they arrive to a class, they have empty stomachs (this is a requirement in order to practice breathing exercises) and often feel cold while wearing additional clothes, like jackets and sweaters. However, during the breathing session, nearly all of them starts to feel warm or even hot. They remove heavy clothes and leave on only T-shirts. This warming effect of breathing exercises on blood sugar levels in overweight people takes place within a few minutes.

With over 30 seconds for the body-O2 test, most people have their nearly ideal weight. (Some people may need up to 50 s to have their ideal weight). Physical exercise becomes more pleasant. Most importantly, they have high levels of energy and improved quality of life.

4.2 Effects of breathing exercises on underweight people

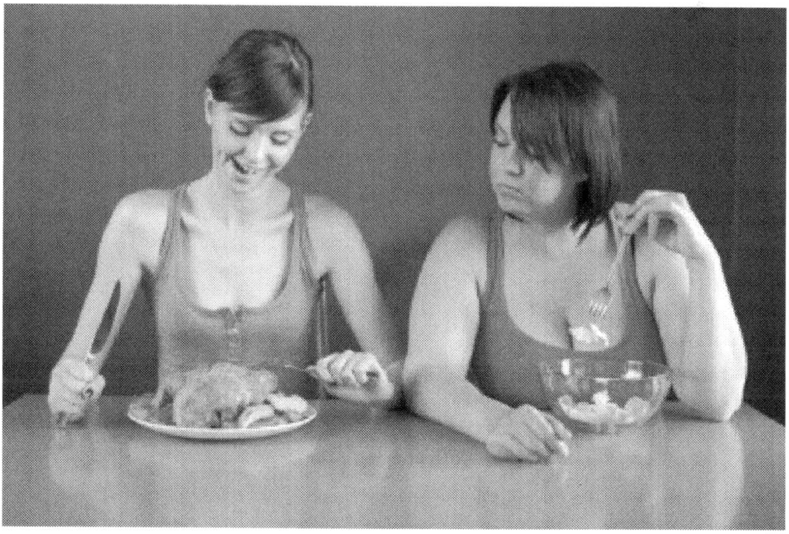

Because of breathing exercises, a small number of people (often due to a poor liver function or some other serious digestive problems) loose weight and become thin. Their chronic hyperventilation makes GI recovery very difficult or impossible. In most serious cases, some of them start to suffer from night sweats and cachexia (as during advanced stages of cancer and HIV-AIDS), when the body triggers catabolic processes, while using proteins and amino-acids as an energy source. Furthermore, due to production of some hormones and/or an abnormal state of the autonomic nervous system, such underweight people often feel warm or hot, with high blood glucose, and have no desire to eat leading to further weight loss. This is another vicious circle where overbreathing plays a central role.

These problems are also possible to solve with breathing retraining and increased CP. The typical effects are as follows. The previously hot or warm underweight person with a high blood glucose level starts to feel colder and hungry immediately after the breathing session. Correct breathing exercises increase blood supply and oxygenation of all digestive organs, including the liver, pancreas, stomach and both intestines. Also, their previously high blood sugar levels drop down due to partial normalization of the metabolism of carbohydrates, lipids and proteins. This is a huge boost in their overall health that allows them to gain weight quickly, often within a few weeks or 2-3 months, and get higher CPs.

Calories generally come from carbohydrates and fats. The common problem is that people with low weight have a weak liver and pancreas, which are able to handle only small amounts of fats and carbohydrates per meal and per day. Apart from low CPs, this also causes problems with weight gain.

The additional solution, apart from the higher CP, for this low-weight problem is too increase honey intake. Raw honey does not require digestive enzymes and is very easy to digest. However, keep in mind that pasteurized honey promotes pathogens in the gut, and one should use only raw (cold pressed or unpasteurized) honey.

Note that honey has some laxative effect due to certain carbohydrates that humans cannot digest. Therefore, it can cause some soiling. However, one does not need to worry about this temporary effect and can use up to 0.5-1 kg of raw honey per day until one's weight is nearly normal, and this feeling of being cold during and after breathing exercises disappears.

Another suggestion is to chew complex carbohydrates or starches very well. (We are going to discuss this topic in more detail later.)

Whatever starchy food someone with low weight eats, from potatoes to bread, rice, corn, and buckwheat, they all should be chewed up to 70-120 times or more until the food disappears in the mouth naturally (without any swallowing movements). This reduces the load on the pancreas since ptyalin and other digestive enzymes from the salivary glands in the mouth can digest up to 80-90% of starches in the mouth. This will help to gain weight fast.

Finally, one can also take steps to restore the liver using betaine hydrochloride (especially if the liver was damaged due to medical drugs or alcohol), black cherry juice (or black cherry juice concentrate), and Milk Thistle (a herb used for liver detoxification that starts to work especially well at over 20 s CP). Use those dosages that are commonly suggested since it is mostly duration of treatment (often 1-3 weeks are required) and especially one's body oxygenation that play the main roles in liver restoration and the appearance of strong hunger or even a voracious appetite.

The first main target for underweight or slim people is about the same: over 20 seconds for the morning CP test.

5. Conclusions and final remarks

As you may notice that this book suggests that science of digestion does not exist yet. Existing books on digestion do not have clear criteria of good (or normal) digestive health and do not provide clear and effective plans to deal with digestive problems.

You can find the detailed recovery plan for people with IBD (Crohn's disease and ulcerative colitis) in part 2 "**Crohn's Disease and Colitis Recovery Guide**" of the same series "**Crohn's Disease and Ulcerative Colitis Books**".

Feel free to leave your questions and comments on the Amazon web page:

http://www.amazon.com/Crohns-Disease-Colitis-Ulcerative-ebook/dp/B009SACFJ2/

and pages devoted to digestive health:

http://www.normalbreathing.com/digestive-health.php

http://www.normalbreathing.com/how-to/how-to-improve-digestion.php

6. Recommended reading

You can also be interested in these books:

Free book (August 2013): "**Jump Start Your Gluten-Free Diet! Living with Celiac / Coeliac Disease & Gluten Intolerance**", by Kim Koeller, Stefano Guandalini MD and Carol Shilson: http://www.amazon.com/Gluten-Free-Coeliac-Intolerance-Allergies-ebook/dp/B00BF1NCM6/

For most people, it is nearly impossible to recover from Crohn's disease or ulcerative colitis, while having bread and other gluten products in diet.

Breaking the Vicious Cycle: Intestinal Health Through Diet
[Paperback only]
by Elaine Gloria Gottschall:
http://www.amazon.com/Breaking-Vicious-Cycle-Intestinal-Through/dp/0969276818/

This is a great book for those who does not have enough time or does not have patience to chew starches very well. Then you can be better without any starches while applying the legendary SCD (special carbohydrate diet).

About the author: Dr. Artour Rakhimov

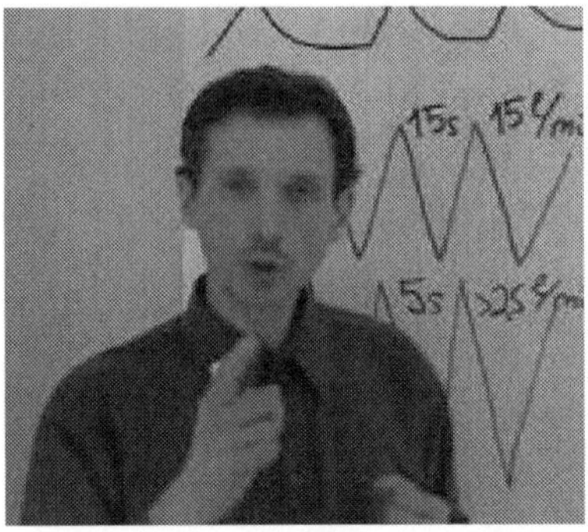

* High School Honor student (Grade "A" for all exams)
* Moscow University Honor student (Grade "A" for all exams)
* Moscow University PhD (Math/Physics), accepted in Canada and the UK
* Winner of many regional competitions in mathematics, chess and sport orienteering (during teenage and University years)
* Good classical piano-player: Chopin, Bach, Tchaikovsky, Beethoven, Strauss (up to now)
* Former captain of the ski-O varsity team and member of the cross-country skiing varsity team of the Moscow State University, best student teams of the USSR
* Former individual coach of world-elite athletes from Soviet (Russian) and Finnish national teams who took gold and silver medals during World Championships
* Total distance covered by running, cross country skiing, and swimming: over 100,000 km or over 2.5 loops around the Earth
* Joined Religious Society of Friends (Quakers) in 2001
* Author of the publication which won Russian National 1998 Contest of scientific and methodological sport papers
* Author of the books, as well as an author of the bestselling Amazon books:
- *"Oxygenate Yourself: Breathe Less" (Buteyko Books; 94 pages; ISBN: 0954599683; 2008; Hardcover)*
- "Cystic Fibrosis Life Expectancy: 30, 50, 70, ..." *2012 - Amazon Kindle book*

- "Doctors Who Cure Cancer" *2012 - Amazon Kindle book*
- "Yoga Benefits Are in Breathing Less" *2012 - Amazon Kindle book*
- "Crohn's Disease and Colitis: Hidden Triggers and Symptoms" *2012 - Amazon Kindle book*
- "How to Use Frolov Breathing Device (Instructions)" *- 2012 - PDF and Amazon book (120 pages)*
- "Amazing DIY Breathing Device" *- 2010-2012 - PDF and Amazon book*
- *"What Science and Professor Buteyko Teach Us About Breathing" 2002*
- *"Breathing, Health and Quality of Life" 2004 (91 pages; Translated in Danish and Finnish)*
- *"Doctor Buteyko Lecture at the Moscow State University" 2009 (55 pages; Translation from Russian with Dr. A. Rakhimov's comments)*
- *"Normal Breathing: the Key to Vital Health" 2009 (The most comprehensive world's book on Buteyko breathing retraining method; over 190,000 words; 305 pages)*

* Author of the world's largest website devoted to breathing, breathing techniques, and breathing retraining (www.NormalBreathing.com)
* Author of numerous YouTube videos (http://www.youtube.com/user/artour2006)
* Buteyko breathing teacher (since 2002 up to now) and trainer
* Inventor of the Amazing DIY breathing device and numerous contributions to breathing retraining
* Whistleblower and investigator of mysterious murder-suicides, massacres and other crimes organized worldwide by GULAG KGB agents using the fast total mind control method
* Practitioner of the New Decision Therapy and Kantillation
* Level 2 Trainer of the New Decision Therapy
* Health writer and health educator

31111421R00044

Made in the USA
Lexington, KY
30 March 2014